THE ULTIMATE CANDIDA DIET COOKBOOK FOR BEGINNERS

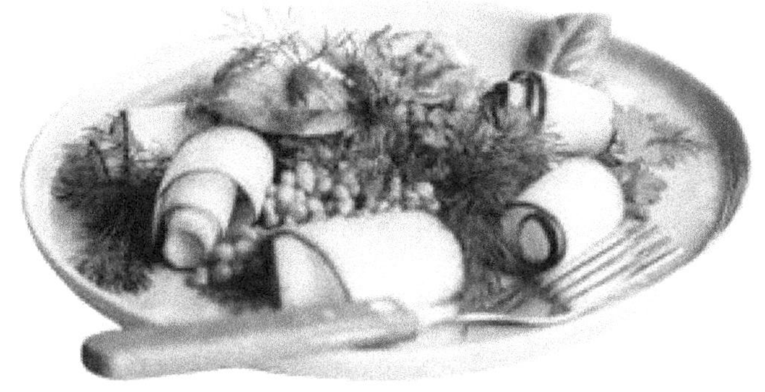

DELICIOUS AND TASTY RECIPES WITH MEAL PLANS TO ALLEVIATE SYMPTOMS, FIGHT YEAST, AND BEAT CANDIDA OVERGROWTH

Dr. Fiona Henry

ADDITIONAL TITLES BY THIS AUTHOR

- ❖ *CANDIDA DIET FOOD LIST*
- ❖ *THE COMPLETE IRON DEFICIENCY ANEMIA COOKBOOK*
- ❖ *MEDITERRANEAN DIET COOKBOOK FOR IRON DEFICIENCY ANEMIA*
- ❖ *OSTEOARTHRITIS DIET COOKBOOK FOR SENIORS*
- ❖ *MEDITERRANEAN DIET COOKBOOK FOR OSTEOARTHRITIS*
- ❖ *MEDITERRANEAN DIET COOKBOOK FOR RHEUMATOID ARTHRITIS*

SCAN THE QR-CODE BELOW

EXTRA BONUS

BONUS

WEEKLY MEAL PLANNER

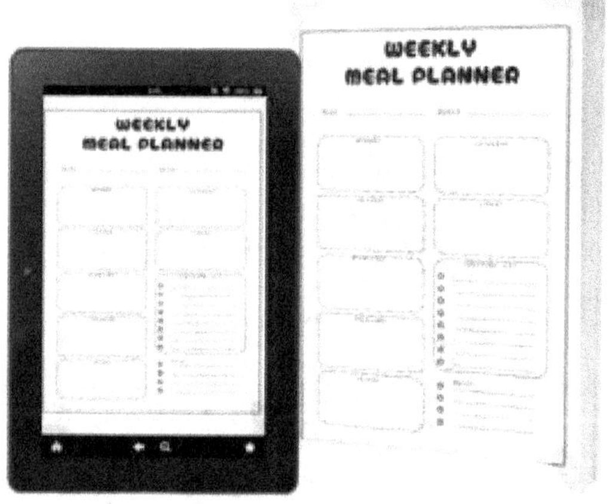

TABLE OF CONTENTS

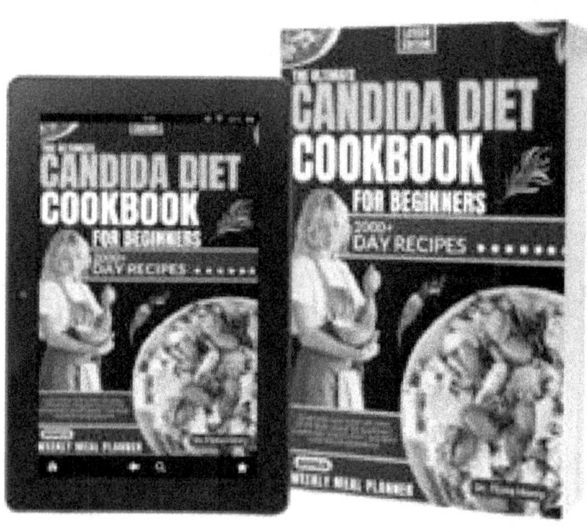

Dear Reader,

Welcome to "The Ultimate Candida Diet Cookbook for Beginners." I am thrilled to introduce myself as Dr. Fiona Henry, a seasoned doctor in the field of nutrition. With years of experience and a passion for helping individuals achieve optimal health through dietary changes, I am excited to bring you this comprehensive guide to managing Candida overgrowth.

In my journey as a nutritionist, I have encountered numerous individuals struggling with various health issues, often stemming from imbalances within the body. Among these challenges, Candida overgrowth stands out as a particularly complex yet often overlooked condition.

Candida, a type of yeast naturally found in the human body, plays a vital role in maintaining a healthy balance of microorganisms in the gut. However, when this delicate balance is disrupted, Candida can proliferate, leading to a range of symptoms and complications.

Understanding Candida overgrowth requires delving into the intricate ecosystem of the human body. As a multifaceted organism, Candida can manifest in various forms, from mild skin irritations to systemic infections affecting multiple organ systems.

Recognizing the signs and symptoms of Candida overgrowth is crucial for early intervention and effective management. From persistent digestive issues to chronic fatigue and recurrent infections, the manifestations of Candida overgrowth can be diverse and often perplexing.

As a dedicated nutritionist, I have witnessed firsthand the transformative power of dietary interventions in combating Candida overgrowth. By addressing underlying dietary factors and implementing targeted meal plans, individuals can significantly alleviate symptoms, restore balance to their gut microbiome, and reclaim their health.

In this comprehensive guide, I aim to provide you with a wealth of knowledge and practical strategies to navigate the challenges posed by Candida overgrowth. From understanding the underlying causes and risk factors to implementing a tailored Candida-friendly diet, each section of this book is designed to empower you on your journey to wellness.

Together, we will explore the fundamental principles of the Candida diet, including foods to avoid and incorporate into your meals, along with invaluable tips for success. Additionally, you will discover a diverse array of delicious and nutritious recipes specifically curated to support your Candida-fighting efforts.

Moreover, I have included a 7-day Candida diet meal plan to help jumpstart your journey and simplify the process of meal preparation. Whether you're seeking nourishing breakfast options, satisfying dinner recipes, or delectable desserts, you'll find a wealth of inspiration within these pages.

I invite you to embark on this transformative journey toward optimal health and vitality. By harnessing the power of nutrition and adopting a Candida-friendly lifestyle, you can take control of your health and conquer Candida overgrowth once and for all.

Candida overgrowth, a condition characterized by the excessive growth of Candida yeast in the body, is a complex and often perplexing health issue that can manifest in various forms. To truly grasp the nuances of Candida overgrowth, it's essential to delve into its fundamental aspects, including its nature, symptoms, causes, management through diet, and available diagnosis and treatment options.

What is Candida?

Candida is a type of yeast that naturally resides in the human body, primarily in the digestive tract, mouth, skin, and reproductive organs. Under normal circumstances, Candida exists in balance with other microorganisms, contributing to the body's overall microbial ecosystem. However, when this balance is disrupted, Candida can proliferate uncontrollably, leading to an overgrowth that can have widespread implications for health.

Signs and Symptoms of Candida Overgrowth

The signs and symptoms of Candida overgrowth can vary widely and may mimic those of other health conditions, making diagnosis challenging. Common manifestations include:

Digestive Issues: Persistent bloating, gas, diarrhea, constipation, and abdominal discomfort are hallmark symptoms of Candida overgrowth. The yeast can disrupt the delicate balance of gut flora, leading to digestive disturbances.

Oral Thrush: Candida overgrowth in the mouth can result in oral thrush, characterized by white patches on the tongue, inner cheeks, roof of the mouth, and throat. When scratched, these patches may bleed and cause pain.

Recurrent Infections: Individuals with Candida overgrowth may experience frequent yeast infections, such as vaginal yeast infections in women or jock itch in men. Additionally, recurrent urinary tract infections (UTIs) may also be associated with Candida overgrowth.

Chronic Fatigue: Fatigue and exhaustion are common complaints among individuals with Candida overgrowth. The body's immune response to the yeast overgrowth can drain energy reserves, leaving individuals feeling persistently tired and lethargic.

Skin Issues: Candida overgrowth can manifest as various skin conditions, including rashes, eczema, psoriasis, and athlete's foot. These skin issues may be accompanied by itching, redness, and inflammation.

Causes and Risk Factors

Candida overgrowth can arise due to a number of circumstances, including:

Antibiotic Use: The indiscriminate use of antibiotics can disrupt the balance of gut flora, creating an environment conducive to Candida overgrowth. Antibiotics eradicate not just pathogenic bacteria but also advantageous microorganisms that aid in controlling Candida.

High Sugar Diet: Excessive consumption of refined sugars and carbohydrates can fuel Candida growth, as yeast thrives on sugar. Diets rich in sugary foods and beverages provide an ideal environment for Candida to flourish.

Weakened Immune System: Individuals with weakened immune systems, such as those with HIV/AIDS, cancer, or autoimmune diseases, are more susceptible to Candida overgrowth. A compromised immune system may struggle to keep Candida in check, allowing it to proliferate unchecked.

Hormonal Imbalances: Fluctuations in hormone levels, such as those seen during pregnancy, menstruation, or hormonal therapy, can predispose individuals to Candida overgrowth. Changes in hormone levels can alter the body's pH balance, creating favorable conditions for yeast growth.

Importance of Diet in Managing Candida

Diet plays a pivotal role in managing Candida overgrowth, as certain foods can either promote or inhibit yeast growth. A Candida-friendly diet focuses on eliminating sugar, refined carbohydrates, and other yeast-promoting foods while emphasizing whole, nutrient-dense foods that support gut health.

Diagnosis and Treatment Options

Diagnosing Candida overgrowth can be challenging due to its varied symptoms and the absence of definitive diagnostic tests. However, healthcare providers may use a combination of medical history, physical examination, laboratory tests, and diagnostic criteria to assess the likelihood of Candida overgrowth.

Treatment for Candida overgrowth typically involves a multifaceted approach aimed at restoring microbial balance, supporting immune function, and addressing underlying dietary and lifestyle factors. Conventional treatment options may include antifungal medications, probiotics, dietary modifications, and lifestyle interventions.

Understanding Candida overgrowth requires a comprehensive exploration of its various facets, from its origins and symptoms to its management through diet and available treatment options. By gaining insight into the complexities of Candida overgrowth, you can take proactive steps to address this pervasive health issue and restore balance to your microbiome.

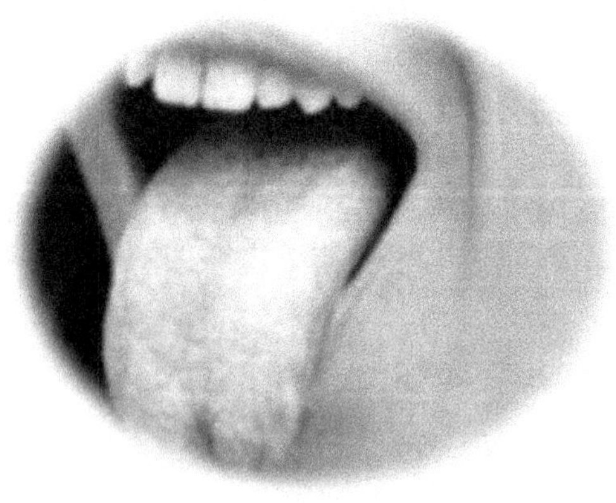

Embarking on the Candida diet marks the beginning of a transformative journey toward restoring balance to your body and reclaiming optimal health. In this section, we will explore the essential components of the Candida diet, including an overview of its principles, key foods to avoid and include, and invaluable tips for success.

Overview of the Candida Diet

The Candida diet is a therapeutic approach designed to rebalance the gut microbiome and inhibit the growth of Candida yeast within the body. By eliminating foods that promote yeast overgrowth and incorporating nutrient-dense, anti-inflammatory foods, the Candida diet aims to create an environment that discourages Candida proliferation and supports overall health.

Foods to Avoid

Central to the Candida diet is the avoidance of foods that can fuel Candida growth and exacerbate symptoms of overgrowth. These include:

Sugar and Sweeteners: Refined sugars, high-fructose corn syrup, and artificial sweeteners provide an ideal fuel source for Candida yeast. Avoid sugary foods and beverages, including desserts, candies, sodas, and sweetened snacks.

Refined Carbohydrates: Processed grains and refined carbohydrates, such as white bread, pasta, and pastries, can spike blood sugar levels and promote yeast overgrowth. Instead, choose complex carbs and healthy grains.

Fruit: While fruits contain natural sugars, some fruits are higher in sugar content and may exacerbate Candida symptoms. Limit or avoid high-sugar fruits such as bananas, grapes, and mangoes, and opt for lower-sugar options like berries and green apples.

Alcohol: Alcohol not only contains sugar but also disrupts gut health and weakens the immune system, making it easier for Candida to proliferate. Eliminate or minimize alcohol consumption, including beer, wine, and spirits.

Dairy: Dairy products can be problematic for individuals with Candida overgrowth due to their lactose content and potential for promoting inflammation. Choose dairy alternatives such as almond milk, coconut milk, or lactose-free options.

Foods to Include

Incorporating nutrient-dense, anti-inflammatory foods is paramount to supporting gut health and combating Candida overgrowth. Focus on including the following foods in your Candida diet:

Non-Starchy Vegetables: Leafy greens, cruciferous vegetables, and other non-starchy vegetables are rich in fiber, vitamins, and minerals while being low in sugar. Aim to include a variety of colorful vegetables in your meals to nourish your body and support detoxification.

Lean Protein: Incorporate lean sources of protein such as poultry, fish, tofu, tempeh, and legumes into your diet to support muscle repair and satiety. Choose organic, pasture-raised, or wild-caught options whenever possible.

Healthy Fats: Include sources of healthy fats such as avocados, nuts, seeds, olive oil, and coconut oil in your diet to provide sustained energy and support hormone balance. These fats also possess anti-inflammatory properties that can aid in combating Candida overgrowth.

Probiotic-Rich Foods: Incorporate fermented foods such as sauerkraut, kimchi, kefir, and yogurt (if tolerated) into your diet to promote a healthy gut microbiome. Probiotics help restore microbial balance and inhibit the growth of Candida yeast.

Tips for Success

Navigating the Candida diet successfully requires dedication, commitment, and a few strategic tips:

Gradual Transition: Ease into the Candida diet gradually to minimize detoxification symptoms and allow your body to adjust to the dietary changes.

Stay Hydrated: Drink plenty of water throughout the day to support detoxification and keep your body hydrated.

Meal Planning: Plan your meals ahead of time and stock up on Candida-friendly ingredients to make meal preparation easier and more convenient.

Supportive Supplements: Consider incorporating supplements such as probiotics, digestive enzymes, and antifungal herbs to complement your Candida diet and support gut health.

Mindful Eating: Practice mindful eating habits, paying attention to hunger and fullness cues, and savoring each bite to enhance digestion and satisfaction.

By implementing these principles and strategies, you can embark on your Candida diet journey with confidence and set yourself up for success in overcoming Candida overgrowth and achieving optimal health.

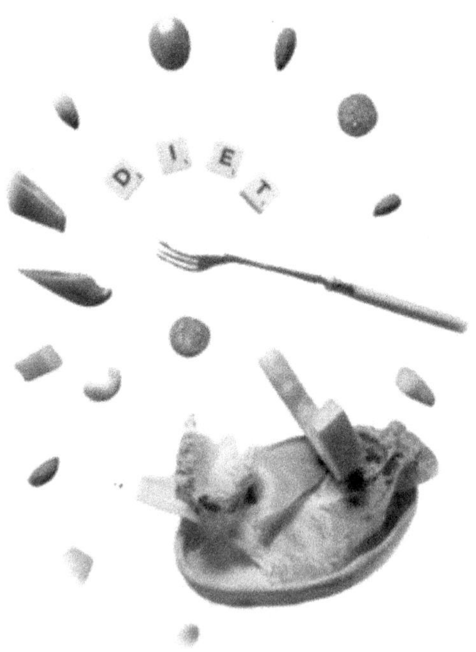

Breakfast Recipes

1. Avocado and Egg Breakfast Bowl

Ingredients:

- 1 ripe avocado, halved and pitted
- 2 eggs
- Salt and pepper to taste
- Optional toppings: cherry tomatoes, sliced cucumber, fresh herbs

Preparation:

1. Preheat the oven to 375°F (190°C).
2. Scoop out a small portion of avocado flesh from each half to create a larger hollow.
3. Crack one egg into each avocado half.
4. Season with salt and pepper.
5. Once the eggs are fried to your preferred doneness, place the avocado halves on a baking sheet and bake for 15 to 20 minutes.
6. Remove from the oven and top with optional toppings if desired.
7. Serve immediately.

Portion Size: 1 avocado half with 1 egg

Cooking Time: 15-20 minutes

Nutritional Information: Approximately 250 calories per serving, rich in healthy fats, protein, and fiber.

2. Coconut Chia Pudding

Ingredients:

- 1/4 cup chia seeds
- 1 cup unsweetened coconut milk
- 1/2 teaspoon vanilla extract
- Optional garnishes include chopped nuts, unsweetened shredded coconut, and fresh berries.

Preparation:

1. In a bowl, mix together chia seeds, coconut milk, and vanilla extract.
2. Stir well to combine, ensuring that the chia seeds are evenly distributed.
3. Cover the bowl and refrigerate overnight, or for at least 4 hours, to allow the chia seeds to absorb the liquid and thicken into pudding.
4. After the pudding has thickened, mix it to distribute the chia seeds.
5. Serve chilled with optional toppings as desired.

Portion Size: 1/2 cup serving

Preparation Time: 5 minutes (plus chilling time)

Nutritional Information: Approximately 180 calories per serving, rich in fiber, healthy fats, and omega-3 fatty acids.

3. Veggie Omelette

Ingredients:

- 2 eggs
- 1/4 cup diced bell peppers (any color)
- 1/4 cup diced onions
- 1/4 cup chopped spinach
- Salt and pepper to taste
- 1 teaspoon olive oil

Preparation:

1. Beat the eggs together in a bowl until thoroughly mixed.
2. In a non-stick skillet, heat the olive oil over medium heat.
3. Add diced bell peppers and onions to the skillet and sauté until softened, about 2-3 minutes.
4. Add chopped spinach to the skillet and cook until wilted, about 1 minute.
5. Pour the beaten eggs over the cooked vegetables in the skillet.
6. Season with salt and pepper.
7. Cook until the edges of the omelette are set, then gently lift the edges and tilt the skillet to allow any uncooked egg to flow underneath.
8. Once the omelette is mostly set, carefully flip it over and cook for an additional 1-2 minutes.
9. Slide the omelette onto a plate and serve hot.

Portion Size: 1 omelette

Cooking Time: 5-7 minutes

Nutritional Information: Approximately 200 calories per serving, rich in protein and essential vitamins and minerals.

4. Almond Flour Pancakes

Ingredients:

- 1 cup almond flour
- 2 eggs
- 1/4 cup unsweetened almond milk
- 1 tablespoon coconut oil, melted
- 1 teaspoon baking powder
- 1/2 teaspoon vanilla extract
- Optional toppings: fresh berries, sugar-free maple syrup, unsweetened shredded coconut

Preparation:

1. In a bowl, whisk together almond flour, eggs, almond milk, melted coconut oil, baking powder, and vanilla extract until smooth.
2. Heat a non-stick skillet or griddle over medium heat and lightly grease with coconut oil.
3. For each pancake, add approximately 1/4 cup of batter to the skillet
4. Cook the pancake until bubbles appear on its surface, then turn it over and continue cooking it until the second side is golden brown.
5. Repeat with the remaining batter.
6. Serve the pancakes hot with optional toppings if desired.

Portion Size: 2-3 pancakes, **Cooking Time:** 5-7 minutes

Nutritional Information: Approximately 250 calories per serving, rich in protein, healthy fats, and fiber.

5. Greek Yogurt Parfait

Ingredients:

- 1/2 cup plain Greek yogurt (unsweetened)
- 1/4 cup fresh berries (such as strawberries, blueberries, or raspberries)
- 1 tablespoon unsweetened shredded coconut
- 1 tablespoon chopped nuts (such as almonds or walnuts)
- Optional: drizzle of sugar-free honey or stevia for sweetness

Preparation:

1. In a glass or bowl, layer Greek yogurt with fresh berries, shredded coconut, and chopped nuts.
2. Continue layering until all the ingredients are utilized.
3. Drizzle with sugar-free honey or sweetener if desired.
4. Serve immediately.

Portion Size: 1 serving

Preparation Time: 5 minutes

Nutritional Information: Approximately 200 calories per serving, rich in protein, probiotics, and antioxidants.

6. Quinoa Breakfast Bowl

Ingredients:

- 1/2 cup cooked quinoa
- 1/4 cup unsweetened almond milk
- 1 tablespoon unsweetened shredded coconut
- 1 tablespoon chopped nuts (such as almonds or walnuts)
- 1/4 teaspoon ground cinnamon
- Optional: drizzle of sugar-free honey or stevia for sweetness

Preparation:

1. In a bowl, combine cooked quinoa with almond milk, shredded coconut, chopped nuts, and ground cinnamon.
2. Stir well to combine.
3. Microwave the quinoa mixture for 1-2 minutes, or until warmed through.
4. Drizzle with sugar-free honey or sweetener if desired.
5. Serve hot.

Portion Size: 1 serving

Preparation Time: 5 minutes

Nutritional Information: Approximately 250 calories per serving, rich in protein, fiber, and essential vitamins and minerals.

7. Smoked Salmon and Avocado Toast

Ingredients:

- 1 slice of whole grain or gluten-free bread
- 1/4 ripe avocado, mashed
- 2 ounces smoked salmon
- Squeeze of fresh lemon juice
- Salt and pepper to taste
- Optional toppings: sliced cucumber, cherry tomatoes, fresh herbs

Preparation:

1. Toast the slice of bread until golden brown.
2. Spread mashed avocado evenly on the toasted bread.
3. Top with smoked salmon.
4. Squeeze fresh lemon juice over the salmon.
5. To taste, add salt and pepper for seasoning.
6. Garnish with optional toppings if desired.
7. Serve immediately.

Portion Size: 1 serving

Preparation Time: 5 minutes

Nutritional Information: Approximately 250 calories per serving, rich in protein, healthy fats, and omega-3 fatty acids.

Nourishing Lunch Recipes

1. Zucchini Noodles with Pesto and Grilled Chicken

Ingredients:

- 2 medium zucchinis, spiralized into noodles
- 1 grilled chicken breast, sliced
- 2 tablespoons homemade or store-bought pesto sauce
- Salt and pepper to taste
- Optional garnish: chopped fresh basil, grated Parmesan cheese

Preparation:

1. Heat a skillet over medium heat and lightly coat with olive oil.
2. Toss in the zucchini noodles and cook for 2 to 3 minutes, or until they are soft
3. Transfer the cooked zucchini noodles to a serving plate.
4. Top with sliced grilled chicken breast.
5. Drizzle pesto sauce over the chicken and zucchini noodles.
6. To taste, add salt and pepper for seasoning.
7. Garnish with chopped fresh basil and grated Parmesan cheese if desired.
8. Serve immediately.

Portion Size: 1 serving

Cooking Time: 10 minutes

Nutritional Information: Approximately 300 calories per serving, rich in protein, fiber, and healthy fats.

2. Quinoa Salad with Lemon-Herb Dressing

Ingredients:

- 1 cup cooked quinoa, cooled
- 1 cup mixed greens (such as spinach, arugula, and kale)
- 1/4 cup cherry tomatoes, halved
- 1/4 cup cucumber, diced
- 1/4 cup bell peppers, diced
- 2 tablespoons chopped fresh herbs (such as parsley, basil, and mint)
- For the dressing:
- 2 tablespoons olive oil
- 1 tablespoon freshly squeezed lemon juice
- 1 teaspoon Dijon mustard
- 1 teaspoon honey or sugar-free sweetener
- Salt and pepper to taste

Preparation:

1. In a large bowl, combine cooked quinoa, mixed greens, cherry tomatoes, cucumber, bell peppers, and chopped fresh herbs.
2. To create the dressing, combine the olive oil, lemon juice, Dijon mustard, honey or other sweetener, salt, and pepper in a small bowl.
3. Pour the dressing over the quinoa salad and toss until well combined.
4. Serve right away or put in the fridge until you're ready to serve.

Portion Size: 1 serving, **Preparation Time:** 15 minutes

Nutritional Information: Approximately 350 calories per serving, rich in protein, fiber, vitamins, and minerals.

3. Salmon and Avocado Salad

Ingredients:

- 4 ounces grilled or baked salmon fillet, flaked
- 1/2 avocado, sliced
- 2 cups mixed salad greens
- 1/4 cup cherry tomatoes, halved
- 1/4 cup cucumber, sliced
- 2 tablespoons sliced red onion
- For the dressing:
- 2 tablespoons olive oil
- 1 tablespoon balsamic vinegar
- 1 teaspoon Dijon mustard
- Salt and pepper to taste

Preparation:

1. Sliced red onion, cucumber, cherry tomatoes, and mixed salad greens should all be combined in a big bowl.
2. Top the salad with flaked salmon and sliced avocado.
3. In a small bowl, whisk together olive oil, balsamic vinegar, Dijon mustard, salt, and pepper to make the dressing.
4. After drizzling the salad with dressing, toss to coat thoroughly.
5. Serve immediately.

Portion Size: 1 serving

Preparation Time: 15 minutes

Nutritional Information: Approximately 350 calories per serving, rich in protein, healthy fats, and antioxidants.

4. Turkey Lettuce Wraps

Ingredients:

- 4 large lettuce leaves (such as romaine or butter lettuce)
- 4 ounces cooked turkey breast, thinly sliced
- 1/4 cup shredded carrots
- 1/4 cup sliced cucumber
- 1/4 cup sliced bell peppers
- 2 tablespoons hummus or tahini
- Optional garnish: chopped fresh herbs, sesame seeds

Preparation:

1. Lay out the lettuce leaves on a flat surface.
2. Divide the sliced turkey breast among the lettuce leaves.
3. Top each lettuce leaf with shredded carrots, sliced cucumber, and bell peppers.
4. Spread hummus or tahini over the turkey and vegetables.
5. To make lettuce wraps, carefully roll up the leaves.
6. Secure with toothpicks if necessary.
7. Serve immediately.

Portion Size: 2 lettuce wraps per serving

Preparation Time: 10 minutes

Nutritional Information: Approximately 200 calories per serving, rich in protein, fiber, and vitamins.

5. Cauliflower Fried Rice

Ingredients:

- Two cups of frozen or fresh cauliflower rice
- 1/4 cup diced carrots
- 1/4 cup diced bell peppers
- 1/4 cup green peas (fresh or frozen)
- 2 green onions, thinly sliced
- 2 eggs, lightly beaten
- Two tablespoons of tamari sauce or coconut amino
- 1 tablespoon sesame oil
- Salt and pepper to taste
- Garnish with sesame seeds and chopped fresh cilantro, if desired.

Preparation:

1. Heat sesame oil in a large skillet or wok over medium heat.
2. Add diced carrots and bell peppers to the skillet and stir-fry for 2-3 minutes until slightly softened.
3. Add cauliflower rice and green peas to the skillet and continue to stir-fry for another 2-3 minutes until heated through.
4. Push the cauliflower rice mixture to one side of the skillet and pour the beaten eggs into the empty space.
5. Scramble the eggs until cooked through, then mix them into the cauliflower rice mixture.
6. Stir in coconut aminos or tamari sauce, sliced green onions, and season with salt and pepper to taste.
7. Cook for an additional 1-2 minutes, then remove from heat.

8. Garnish with chopped fresh cilantro and sesame seeds if desired.
9. Serve hot.

Portion Size: 1 serving

Cooking Time: 15 minutes

Nutritional Information: Approximately 250 calories per serving, rich in fiber, protein, and vitamins.

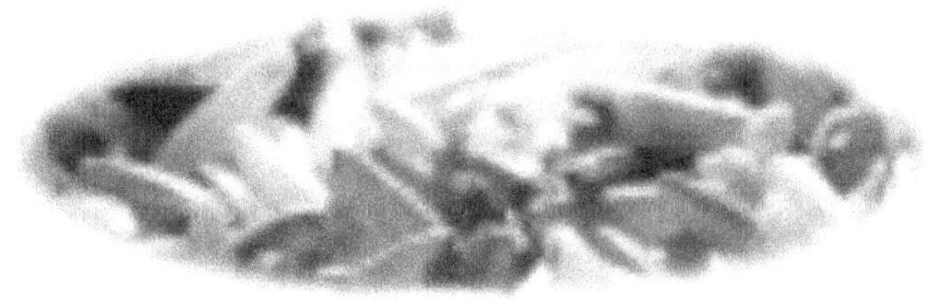

6. Lentil and Vegetable Soup

Ingredients:

- 1/2 cup rinsed and drained dried lentils, either brown or green
- 2 cups vegetable broth
- 1 cup diced tomatoes (fresh or canned)
- 1/2 cup diced carrots
- 1/2 cup diced celery
- 1/4 cup diced onion
- 2 cloves garlic, minced
- 1 teaspoon ground cumin
- 1/2 teaspoon ground turmeric
- Salt and pepper to taste
- Optional garnish: chopped fresh parsley or cilantro

Preparation:

1. In a large pot, combine lentils, vegetable broth, diced tomatoes, carrots, celery, onion, garlic, cumin, turmeric, salt, and pepper.
2. Bring the mixture to a boil over medium-high heat, then reduce heat to low and simmer for 20-25 minutes until the lentils and vegetables are tender.
3. Adjust seasoning with additional salt and pepper if needed.
4. Ladle the soup into bowls and garnish with chopped fresh parsley or cilantro if desired.
5. Serve hot.

Portion Size: 1 serving, **Cooking Time:** 25 minutes

Nutritional Information: Approximately 300 calories per serving, rich in fiber, protein, and essential nutrients.

<u>7. Tuna Salad Stuffed Bell Peppers</u>

Ingredients:

- Two large bell peppers, seeded and half
- One can (5 ounces) of drained tuna in water
- 1/4 cup diced celery
- 1/4 cup diced red onion
- 2 tablespoons plain Greek yogurt (unsweetened)
- 1 tablespoon Dijon mustard
- Salt and pepper to taste
- Optional garnish: sliced avocado, chopped fresh parsley

Preparation:

1. Preheat the oven to 375°F (190°C).
2. Place bell pepper halves on a baking sheet lined with parchment paper.
3. In a bowl, combine drained tuna, diced celery, diced red onion, Greek yogurt, Dijon mustard, salt, and pepper.
4. Mix well to combine.
5. Spoon the tuna salad mixture into each bell pepper half.
6. Bake in the preheated oven for 20-25 minutes until the bell peppers are tender.
7. Remove from the oven and garnish with sliced avocado and chopped fresh parsley if desired.
8. Serve hot or cold.

Portion Size: 2 stuffed pepper halves per serving, **Cooking Time:** 25 minutes

Nutritional Information: Approximately 250 calories per serving, rich in protein, fiber, and healthy fats.

1. Lemon Herb Baked Salmon

Ingredients:

- Two fillets of salmon (approximately 4-6 ounces each)
- 2 tablespoons olive oil
- 1 tablespoon freshly squeezed lemon juice
- 1 clove garlic, minced
- 1 teaspoon dried thyme
- 1 teaspoon dried oregano
- Salt and pepper to taste
- Lemon slices for garnish

Preparation:

1. Before proceeding, preheat the oven to 375°F (190°C) and place parchment paper on a baking pan.
2. In a small bowl, whisk together olive oil, lemon juice, minced garlic, dried thyme, dried oregano, salt, and pepper.
3. After the baking sheet is ready, put the salmon fillets on it.
4. Brush the lemon herb mixture over the salmon fillets, ensuring they are evenly coated.
5. Place a lemon slice on top of each salmon fillet for extra flavor.
6. Bake the salmon for 12 to 15 minutes, or until it is cooked through and flake readily with a fork, in an oven that has been warmed.
7. Serve hot with your choice of side dishes.

Portion Size: 1 salmon fillet per serving,

Cooking Time: 15 minutes

Nutritional Information: Approximately 300-400 calories per serving, rich in protein, omega-3 fatty acids, and essential nutrients.

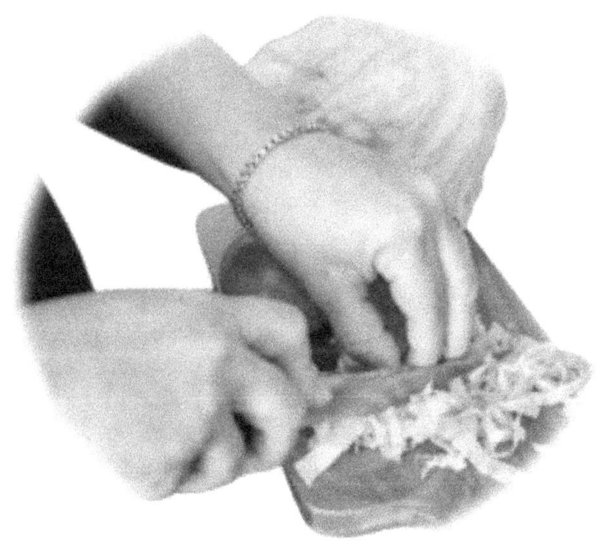

2. Grilled Lemon Garlic Chicken

Ingredients:

- 2 boneless, skinless chicken breasts
- 2 tablespoons olive oil
- 2 tablespoons freshly squeezed lemon juice
- 2 cloves garlic, minced
- 1 teaspoon dried oregano
- Salt and pepper to taste
- Fresh parsley for garnish

Preparation:

1. In a bowl, whisk together olive oil, lemon juice, minced garlic, dried oregano, salt, and pepper to make the marinade.
2. Place the chicken breasts in a shallow dish and pour the marinade over them, ensuring they are evenly coated.
3. Cover the dish and marinate the chicken in the refrigerator for at least 30 minutes, or up to 4 hours.
4. Preheat the grill to medium-high heat.
5. Remove the chicken from the marinade and discard any excess marinade.
6. Grill the chicken breasts for 6-8 minutes per side, or until they are cooked through and have grill marks.
7. Transfer the grilled chicken to a serving platter and garnish with fresh parsley.
8. Warm up and serve with your preferred side dishes.

Portion Size: 1 chicken breast per serving,

Cooking Time: 15 minutes (plus marinating time)

Nutritional Information: Approximately 250-300 calories per serving, rich in protein, low in carbohydrates.

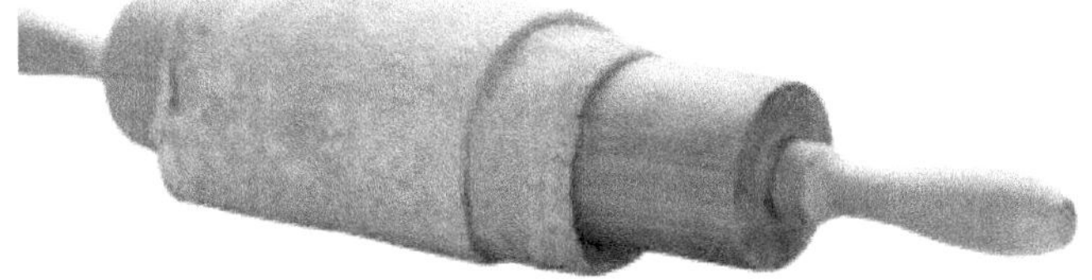

3. Cauliflower Rice Stir-Fry

Ingredients:

- Two cups of frozen or fresh cauliflower rice
- 1 cup mixed vegetables (such as bell peppers, carrots, broccoli, snap peas)
- 1/4 cup diced onion
- 2 cloves garlic, minced
- Two tablespoons of tamari sauce or coconut aminos
- 1 tablespoon sesame oil
- Salt and pepper to taste
- Optional protein: cooked shrimp, chicken, tofu, or tempeh

Preparation:

1. Heat sesame oil in a large skillet or wok over medium heat.
2. Add diced onion and minced garlic to the skillet and sauté for 2-3 minutes until fragrant.
3. Add mixed vegetables to the skillet and stir-fry for 5-7 minutes until tender-crisp.
4. Push the vegetables to one side of the skillet and add cauliflower rice to the empty space.
5. Stir-fry the cauliflower rice for 3-4 minutes until heated through.
6. Mix the cauliflower rice with the cooked vegetables in the skillet.
7. Add coconut aminos or tamari sauce to the skillet and toss until everything is well coated.
8. To taste, add salt and pepper for seasoning.

9. If desired, add cooked protein such as shrimp, chicken, tofu, or tempeh to the skillet and toss to combine.
10. Serve hot as a standalone dish or with your choice of protein.

Portion Size: 1-2 cups per serving

Cooking Time: 15 minutes

Nutritional Information: Approximately 150-200 calories per serving, rich in fiber, vitamins, and minerals.

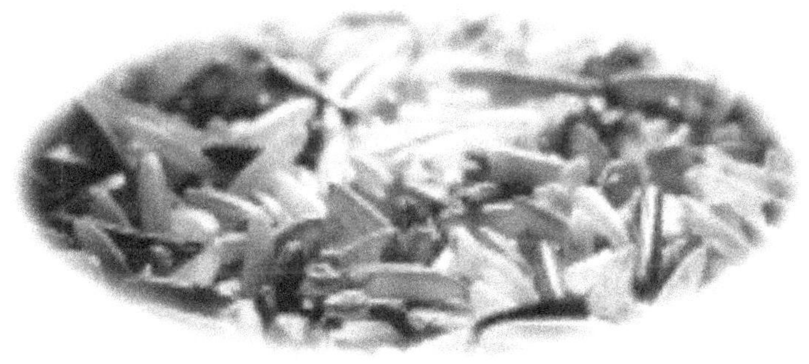

4. Turkey and Vegetable Stir-Fry

Ingredients:

- 8 ounces lean ground turkey
- 2 cups mixed vegetables (such as bell peppers, zucchini, mushrooms, snow peas)
- 1/4 cup diced onion
- 2 cloves garlic, minced
- Two tablespoons of tamari sauce or coconut aminos
- 1 tablespoon sesame oil
- Salt and pepper to taste
- Optional garnish: sliced green onions, sesame seeds

Preparation:

1. Heat sesame oil in a large skillet or wok over medium heat.
2. Add diced onion and minced garlic to the skillet and sauté for 2-3 minutes until fragrant.
3. Add ground turkey to the skillet and cook until browned and cooked through, breaking it up with a spatula.
4. Add mixed vegetables to the skillet and stir-fry for 5-7 minutes until tender-crisp.
5. Pour coconut aminos or tamari sauce over the turkey and vegetables in the skillet.
6. Stir to combine and season with salt and pepper to taste.
7. Cook for a further two to three minutes, or until well heated.
8. If preferred, garnish with sesame seeds and sliced green onions.

9. Serve hot as a standalone dish or with cauliflower rice or quinoa.

Portion Size: 1-2 cups per serving

Cooking Time: 20 minutes

Nutritional Information: Approximately 200-300 calories per serving, rich in protein, fiber, and essential nutrients.

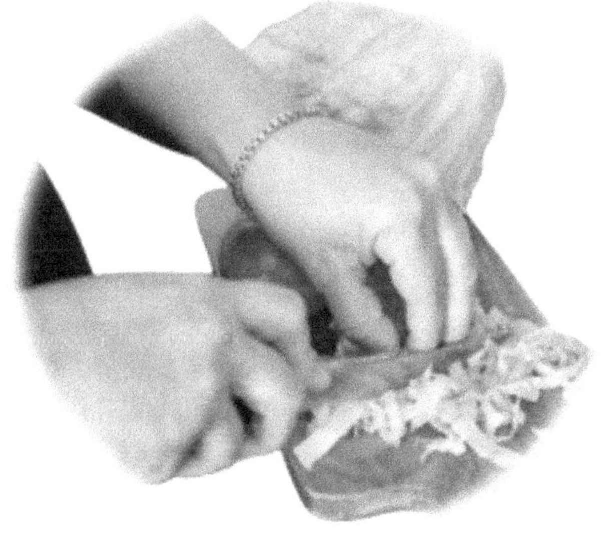

5. Baked Stuffed Bell Peppers

Ingredients:

- Two large bell peppers, seeded and half
- 1 cup cooked quinoa or cauliflower rice
- 1 cup cooked black beans
- 1/2 cup diced tomatoes
- 1/4 cup diced onion
- 2 cloves garlic, minced
- 1 teaspoon ground cumin
- 1/2 teaspoon chili powder
- Salt and pepper to taste
- Optional toppings: shredded cheese, chopped fresh cilantro, sliced avocado

Preparation:

1. Preheat the oven to 375°F (190°C) and line a baking dish with parchment paper.
2. In a bowl, combine cooked quinoa or cauliflower rice, cooked black beans, diced tomatoes, diced onion, minced garlic, ground cumin, chili powder, salt, and pepper.
3. Mix well to combine.
4. Fill each bell pepper half with the quinoa or cauliflower rice mixture, pressing down gently to pack it in.
5. Place the stuffed bell peppers in the prepared baking dish.
6. Cover the dish with foil and bake in the preheated oven for 25-30 minutes, or until the peppers are tender.

7. Remove the foil and sprinkle shredded cheese over the stuffed bell peppers if desired.
8. Return the baking dish to the oven and bake for an additional 5 minutes, or until the cheese is melted and bubbly.
9. Garnish with chopped fresh cilantro and sliced avocado if desired.
10. Serve hot as a standalone dish or with a side salad.

Portion Size: 1-2 stuffed pepper halves per serving

Cooking Time: 35 minutes

Nutritional Information: Approximately 300-400 calories per serving, rich in protein, fiber, and essential vitamins and minerals.

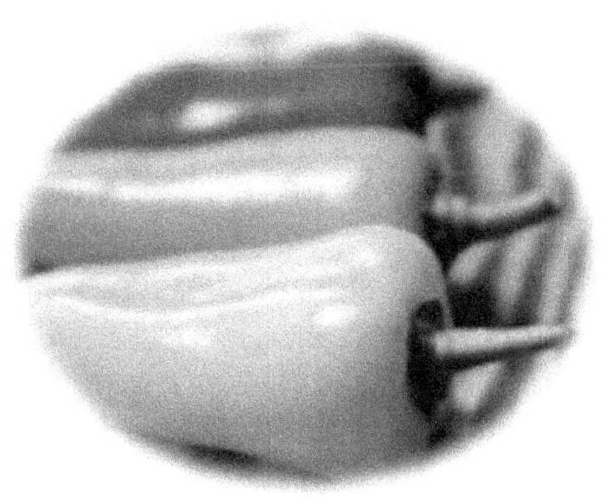

6. Eggplant and Zucchini Lasagna

Ingredients:

- One big eggplant cut into thin slices lengthwise
- 2 small zucchinis, sliced lengthwise into thin strips
- 1 cup marinara sauce (sugar-free)
- 1 cup ricotta cheese (or dairy-free alternative)
- 1/2 cup shredded mozzarella cheese (or dairy-free alternative)
- Two tablespoons of nutritional yeast or grated Parmesan cheese
- 1 teaspoon dried basil
- 1 teaspoon dried oregano
- Salt and pepper to taste
- Fresh basil leaves for garnish

Preparation:

1. Preheat the oven to 375°F (190°C) and lightly grease a baking dish.
2. Lay half of the eggplant slices in the bottom of the prepared baking dish, slightly overlapping.
3. Spread half of the marinara sauce over the eggplant slices.
4. In a bowl, combine ricotta cheese, shredded mozzarella cheese, grated Parmesan cheese, dried basil, dried oregano, salt, and pepper.
5. Spread half of the ricotta cheese mixture over the marinara sauce layer.
6. Repeat the layers with the remaining zucchini slices, marinara sauce, and ricotta cheese mixture.
7. Cover the baking dish with foil and bake in the preheated oven for 30-35 minutes, or until the

vegetables are tender and the cheese is melted and bubbly.
8. Remove the foil and bake for an additional 5 minutes to brown the cheese slightly.
9. Garnish with fresh basil leaves before serving.
10. Before slicing and serving, allow the lasagna to cool for a few minutes.

Portion Size: 1-2 slices per serving

Cooking Time: 40 minutes

Nutritional Information: Approximately 300-400 calories per serving, rich in protein, fiber, and calcium.

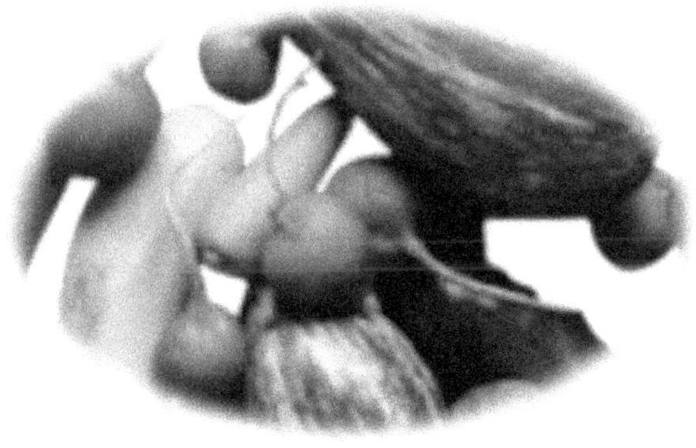

7. Coconut Curry Shrimp

Ingredients:

- 8 ounces shrimp, peeled and deveined
- 1 tablespoon coconut oil
- 1 small onion, diced
- 2 cloves garlic, minced
- 1 tablespoon grated ginger
- 1 tablespoon curry powder
- 1 can (14 ounces) coconut milk (full-fat)
- One cup of mixed veggies, including carrots, snap peas, and bell
- Salt and pepper to taste
- Fresh cilantro for garnish

Preparation:

1. Heat the coconut oil in a big skillet over medium heat.
2. Add diced onion, minced garlic, and grated ginger to the skillet and sauté for 2-3 minutes until fragrant.
3. After adding the curry powder, simmer for an additional minute.
4. Add coconut milk to the skillet and bring to a simmer.
5. Add mixed vegetables to the skillet and cook for 5-7 minutes until tender.
6. Add shrimp to the skillet and cook for 2-3 minutes until pink and cooked through.
7. Season with salt and pepper to taste.
8. Garnish with fresh cilantro before serving.
9. Serve hot over cooked quinoa or cauliflower rice.

Portion Size: 1 serving

Cooking Time: 20 minutes

Nutritional Information: Approximately 300-400 calories per serving, rich in protein, healthy fats, and fiber.

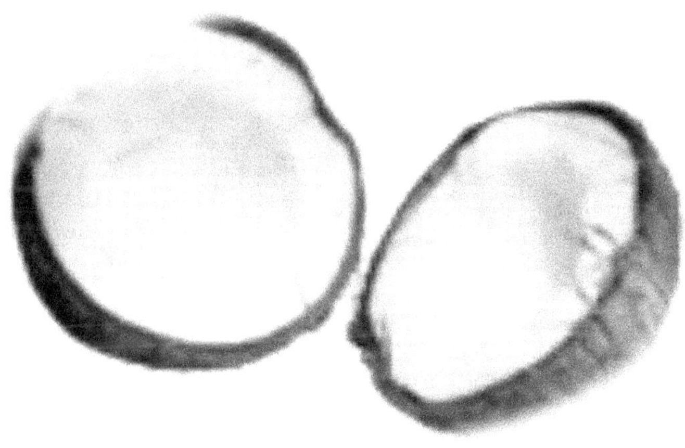

1. Cucumber Avocado Salad

Ingredients:

- 1 large cucumber, diced
- 1 ripe avocado, diced
- 1 tablespoon lemon juice
- 1 tablespoon olive oil
- 1 tablespoon chopped fresh cilantro
- Salt and pepper to taste

Preparation:

1. In a bowl, combine diced cucumber and avocado.
2. Drizzle lemon juice and olive oil over the cucumber and avocado.
3. Add chopped cilantro, salt, and pepper to taste.
4. Toss gently to combine all ingredients.
5. Serve chilled as a refreshing snack or side dish.

Portion Size: 1 serving

Preparation Time: 5 minutes

Nutritional Information: Approximately 150 calories per serving, rich in healthy fats, fiber, vitamins, and minerals.

2. Roasted Garlic Hummus

Ingredients:

- One can (15 ounces) of rinsed and drained chickpeas
- 2 cloves garlic, roasted
- 2 tablespoons tahini
- 2 tablespoons lemon juice
- 1 tablespoon olive oil
- 1/4 teaspoon ground cumin
- Salt and pepper to taste
- Water (as needed for consistency)

Preparation:

1. Preheat the oven to 400°F (200°C).
2. Wrap garlic cloves in aluminum foil and roast in the oven for 20-25 minutes, or until soft and fragrant.
3. In a food processor, combine chickpeas, roasted garlic, tahini, lemon juice, olive oil, ground cumin, salt, and pepper.
4. Process until smooth, adding water as needed to reach desired consistency.
5. Adjust seasoning to taste.
6. Transfer the hummus to a serving bowl and drizzle with a little extra olive oil.
7. Serve with raw vegetable sticks or whole grain crackers as a healthy snack or side dish.

Portion Size: 2 tablespoons per serving

Preparation Time: 30 minutes (including roasting time)

Nutritional Information: Approximately 70 calories per serving, rich in protein, fiber, healthy fats, and antioxidants.

3. Baked Sweet Potato Fries

Ingredients:

- 2 medium sweet potatoes, peeled and cut into fries
- 1 tablespoon olive oil
- 1 teaspoon paprika
- 1/2 teaspoon garlic powder
- 1/2 teaspoon onion powder
- Salt and pepper to taste

Preparation:

1. Adjust the oven temperature to 425°F (220°C) and place parchment paper on a baking pan.
2. In a bowl, toss sweet potato fries with olive oil, paprika, garlic powder, onion powder, salt, and pepper until evenly coated.
3. Spread the fries in a single layer on the prepared baking sheet.
4. Bake in the preheated oven for 20-25 minutes, flipping halfway through, until the fries are golden brown and crispy.
5. Remove from the oven and serve hot as a satisfying snack or side dish.

Portion Size: 1 serving

Cooking Time: 25 minutes

Nutritional Information: Approximately 150 calories per serving, rich in fiber, vitamins, and minerals.

4. Zucchini Chips

Ingredients:

- 2 medium zucchinis, thinly sliced
- 1 tablespoon olive oil
- 1/2 teaspoon garlic powder
- 1/2 teaspoon onion powder
- 1/4 teaspoon paprika
- Salt and pepper to taste

Preparation:

1. Preheat the oven to 225°F (110°C) and line a baking sheet with parchment paper.
2. In a bowl, toss zucchini slices with olive oil, garlic powder, onion powder, paprika, salt, and pepper until evenly coated.
3. Arrange the zucchini slices in a single layer on the prepared baking sheet.
4. Bake in the preheated oven for 2-3 hours, flipping halfway through, until the zucchini chips are crisp and golden brown.
5. Before serving, take out of the oven and allow it cool.
6. Enjoy as a crunchy and flavorful snack or side dish.

Portion Size: 1 serving

Cooking Time: 2-3 hours

Nutritional Information: Approximately 100 calories per serving, rich in fiber, vitamins, and antioxidants.

5. Guacamole with Veggie Sticks

Ingredients:

- 2 ripe avocados, peeled and mashed
- 1 small tomato, diced
- 1/4 cup diced red onion
- 1/4 cup chopped fresh cilantro
- 1 tablespoon lime juice
- Salt and pepper to taste
- Assorted vegetable sticks (such as carrots, celery, bell peppers) for dipping

Preparation:

1. Mash avocados, diced tomatoes, diced red onions, chopped cilantro, lime juice, salt, and pepper should all be combined in a bowl.
2. Mix well to combine all ingredients.
3. Serve the guacamole with assorted vegetable sticks for dipping.
4. Enjoy as a nutritious and satisfying snack or side dish.

Portion Size: 1 serving

Preparation Time: 10 minutes

Nutritional Information: Approximately 150 calories per serving, rich in healthy fats, fiber, vitamins, and minerals.

6. Cabbage Slaw with Apple Cider Vinegar Dressing

Ingredients:

- 2 cups shredded green cabbage
- 1/2 cup shredded carrots
- 1/4 cup diced red onion
- 2 tablespoons apple cider vinegar
- 1 tablespoon olive oil
- 1 teaspoon honey or sugar-free sweetener
- Salt and pepper to taste

Preparation:

1. In a large bowl, combine shredded cabbage, shredded carrots, and diced red onion.
2. In a small bowl, whisk together apple cider vinegar, olive oil, honey or sweetener, salt, and pepper to make the dressing.
3. After pouring the dressing over the cabbage mixture, toss to coat thoroughly.
4. Let the slaw marinate in the refrigerator for at least 30 minutes before serving.
5. Serve chilled as a refreshing snack or side dish.

Portion Size: 1 serving

Preparation Time: 10 minutes (plus marinating time)

Nutritional Information: Approximately 100 calories per serving, rich in fiber, vitamins, and antioxidants.

7. Greek Yogurt with Berries

Ingredients:

- 1/2 cup plain Greek yogurt (unsweetened)
- 1/4 cup mixed berries (such as strawberries, blueberries, raspberries)
- 1 tablespoon unsweetened shredded coconut
- One tablespoon of finely chopped nuts (walnuts, almonds, etc.)
- Optional: drizzle of honey or sugar-free sweetener for sweetness

Preparation:

1. In a bowl, layer Greek yogurt with mixed berries, shredded coconut, and chopped nuts.
2. Drizzle with honey or sweetener if desired.
3. Serve immediately as a satisfying snack or side dish.

Portion Size: 1 serving

Preparation Time: 5 minutes

Nutritional Information: Approximately 150 calories per serving, rich in protein, probiotics, fiber, and antioxidants.

1. Coconut Chia Pudding

Ingredients:

- 1/4 cup chia seeds
- 1 cup coconut milk (unsweetened)
- 1 tablespoon maple syrup or sugar-free sweetener
- 1/2 teaspoon vanilla extract
- Fresh berries for garnish

Preparation:

1. In a bowl, whisk together chia seeds, coconut milk, maple syrup or sweetener, and vanilla extract.
2. Cover the bowl and refrigerate for at least 2 hours or overnight, until the mixture thickens and sets.
3. Stir the pudding before serving to ensure an even consistency.
4. Divide the pudding into serving cups and top with fresh berries.
5. Serve chilled as a satisfying and creamy dessert option.

Portion Size: 1 serving

Preparation Time: 5 minutes (plus chilling time)

Nutritional Information: Approximately 200 calories per serving, rich in fiber, healthy fats, and antioxidants.

2. Baked Cinnamon Apple Slices

Ingredients:

- 2 apples, cored and thinly sliced
- 1 tablespoon coconut oil, melted
- 1 teaspoon ground cinnamon
- 1/2 teaspoon ground nutmeg
- 1/4 teaspoon ground cloves
- Optional: drizzle of honey or sugar-free sweetener

Preparation:

1. Preheat the oven to 350°F (180°C) and line a baking sheet with parchment paper.
2. In a bowl, toss apple slices with melted coconut oil, ground cinnamon, ground nutmeg, and ground cloves until evenly coated.
3. Spread the apple slices in a single layer on the prepared baking sheet.
4. Bake in the preheated oven for 15-20 minutes, or until the apples are soft and slightly caramelized.
5. Take out of the oven and allow it to cool down a little before serving.
6. Drizzle with honey or sweetener if desired.
7. Serve warm as a comforting and aromatic dessert option.

Portion Size: 1 serving

Cooking Time: 20 minutes

Nutritional Information: Approximately 150 calories per serving, rich in fiber, vitamins, and antioxidants.

3. Avocado Chocolate Mousse

Ingredients:

- 1 ripe avocado, peeled and pitted
- 2 tablespoons unsweetened cocoa powder
- 2 tablespoons maple syrup or sugar-free sweetener
- 1/2 teaspoon vanilla extract
- Pinch of salt
- Optional toppings: sliced strawberries, chopped nuts

Preparation:

1. Ripe avocado, cocoa powder, vanilla extract, maple syrup or other sweetener, and a dash of salt should all be combined in a food processor or blender.
2. Blend until smooth and creamy, scraping down the sides as needed.
3. Taste and adjust sweetness if necessary by adding more maple syrup or sweetener.
4. Transfer the avocado chocolate mousse to serving bowls or glasses.
5. Before serving, let the food cool for at least half an hour in the refrigerator.
6. Garnish with sliced strawberries and chopped nuts if desired.
7. Serve chilled as a decadent and indulgent dessert option.

Portion Size: 1 serving

Preparation Time: 10 minutes (plus chilling time)

Nutritional Information: Approximately 200 calories per serving, rich in healthy fats, fiber, and antioxidants.

4. Lemon Coconut Energy Balls

Ingredients:

- 1 cup unsweetened shredded coconut
- 1/2 cup almond flour
- 1/4 cup coconut oil, melted
- 2 tablespoons honey or sugar-free sweetener
- Zest and juice of 1 lemon
- Pinch of salt

Preparation:

1. In a food processor, combine shredded coconut, almond flour, melted coconut oil, honey or sweetener, lemon zest, lemon juice, and a pinch of salt.
2. Pulse until the mixture comes together and forms a dough-like consistency.
3. Roll the dough into small balls using your hands.
4. Transfer the energy balls to a parchment paper-lined plate or baking sheet.
5. Chill in the refrigerator for at least 30 minutes to firm up.
6. Store the energy balls in an airtight container in the refrigerator until ready to serve.
7. Enjoy as a nutritious and energizing snack or dessert option.

Portion Size: 1-2 energy balls per serving

Preparation Time: 15 minutes (plus chilling time)

Nutritional Information: Approximately 100 calories per serving, rich in healthy fats, fiber, and natural sugars.

5. Berry Coconut Yogurt Parfait

Ingredients:

- 1 cup unsweetened coconut yogurt
- Half a cup of mixed berries, including raspberries, blueberries, and strawberries
- 2 tablespoons unsweetened shredded coconut
- 2 tablespoons chopped nuts (such as almonds, walnuts)
- Optional: drizzle of honey or sugar-free sweetener

Preparation:

1. In a glass or serving bowl, layer coconut yogurt with mixed berries, shredded coconut, and chopped nuts.
2. Drizzle with honey or sweetener if desired.
3. Repeat the layers until the glass or bowl is filled.
4. Serve immediately as a refreshing and creamy dessert option.

Portion Size: 1 serving

Preparation Time: 5 minutes

Nutritional Information: Approximately 200 calories per serving, rich in probiotics, fiber, vitamins, and antioxidants.

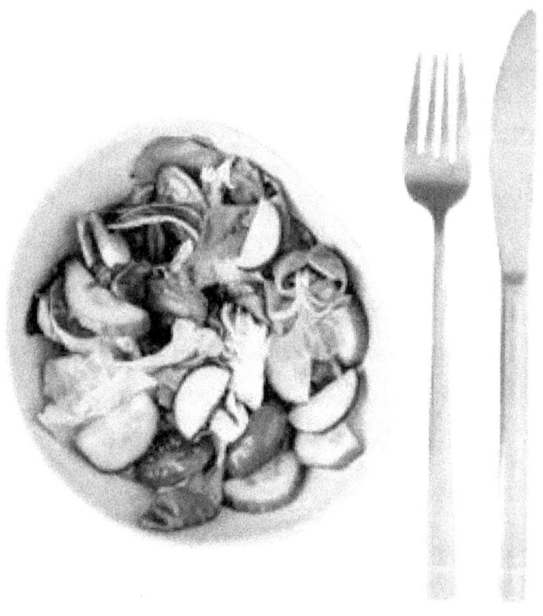

DAY 1

BREAKFAST: **Avocado and Egg Breakfast Bowl**

LUNCH: **Zucchini Noodles with Pesto and Grilled Chicken**

DINNER: **Lemon Herb Baked Salmon**

SNACK: **Cucumber Avocado Salad**

DESSERT: **Baked Cinnamon Apple Slices**

DAY 2

BREAKFAST: **Coconut Chia Pudding**

LUNCH: **Quinoa Salad with Lemon-Herb Dressing**

DINNER: **Grilled Lemon Garlic Chicken**

SNACK: **Roasted Garlic Hummus**

DESSERT: **Coconut Chia Pudding**

DAY 3

BREAKFAST: **Veggie Omelette**

LUNCH: **Salmon and Avocado Salad**

DINNER: **Cauliflower Rice Stir-Fry**

SNACK: **Baked Sweet Potato Fries**

DESSERT: **Berry Coconut Yogurt Parfait**

DAY 4

BREAKFAST: **Almond Flour Pancakes**

LUNCH: **Turkey Lettuce Wraps**

DINNER: **Turkey and Vegetable Stir-Fry**

SNACK: **Zucchini Chips**

DESSERT: **Lemon Coconut Energy Balls**

DAY 5

BREAKFAST: **Greek Yogurt Parfait**

LUNCH: **Cauliflower Fried Rice**

DINNER: **Baked Stuffed Bell Peppers**

SNACK: **Guacamole with Veggie Sticks**

DESSERT: **Avocado Chocolate Mousse**

DAY 6

BREAKFAST: **Quinoa Breakfast Bowl**

LUNCH: **Lentil and Vegetable Soup**

DINNER: **Eggplant and Zucchini Lasagna**

SNACK: **Cabbage Slaw with Apple Cider Vinegar Dressing**

DESSERT: **Baked Cinnamon Apple Slices**

BREAKFAST: **Smoked Salmon and Avocado Toast**

LUNCH: **Tuna Salad Stuffed Bell Peppers**

DINNER: **Coconut Curry Shrimp**

SNACK: **Greek Yogurt with Berries**

DESSERT: **Coconut Chia Pudding**

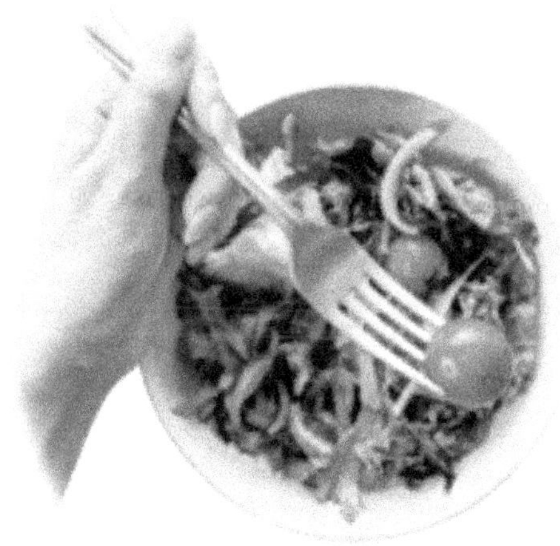

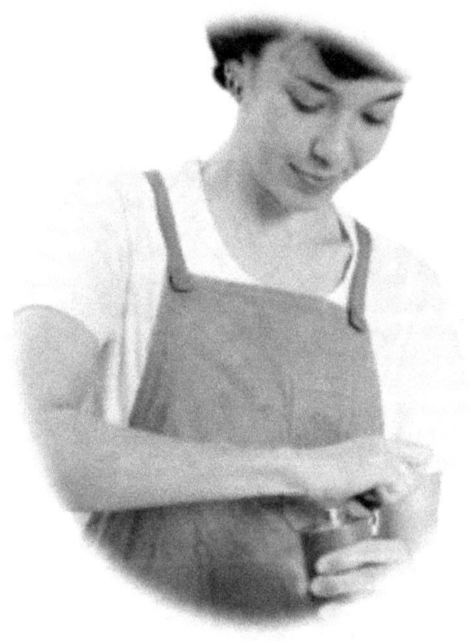

CONCLUSION

Throughout this cookbook, we have explored the fundamentals of understanding Candida overgrowth, including its causes, symptoms, and the crucial role of diet in managing this condition.

By providing a variety of quick and easy recipes for breakfast, lunch, dinner, snacks, and desserts, we aim to empower you with delicious and Candida-friendly options that not only nourish the body but also support overall health and well-being. Each recipe is thoughtfully crafted with Candida-friendly ingredients and accompanied by detailed nutritional information, cooking instructions, and portion sizes to help you make informed dietary choices.

Whether you are just beginning your journey to combat Candida overgrowth or seeking inspiration for flavorful and wholesome meals, this cookbook serves as a valuable resource to guide you towards a healthier lifestyle. We encourage you to explore these recipes, experiment with different flavors and ingredients, and discover the joy of eating well while supporting your body's natural balance.

With dedication, patience, and the right tools at your disposal, overcoming Candida overgrowth is within reach. Embrace the power of nutritious and delicious foods, and take proactive steps towards reclaiming your health and vitality.

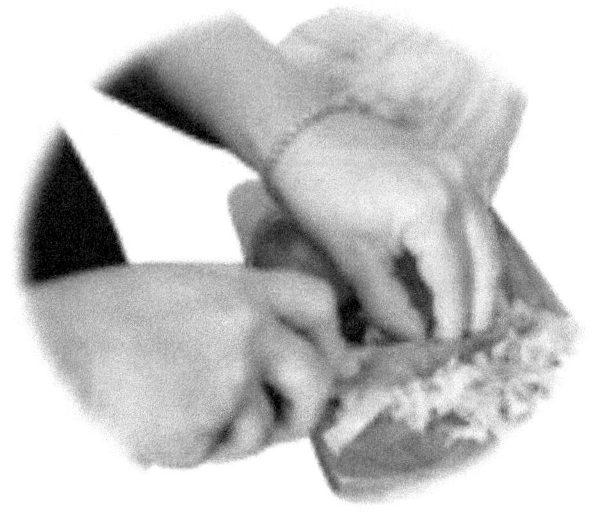

Here's to your journey towards wellness and vitality with the help of "The Candida Diet Cookbook for Beginners."

WEEKLY MEAL PLANNER

WEEK ___________________   MONTH ___________________

MONDAY

SATURDAY

TUESDAY

SUNDAY

WEDNESDAY

SHOPPING LIST

THURSDAY

FRIDAY

NOTES:

WEEKLY MEAL PLANNER

WEEK _______________   MONTH _______________

MONDAY

SATURDAY

TUESDAY

SUNDAY

WEDNESDAY

SHOPPING LIST

THURSDAY

FRIDAY

NOTES:

WEEKLY MEAL PLANNER

WEEK ___________________   MONTH ___________________

MONDAY

TUESDAY

WEDNESDAY

THURSDAY

FRIDAY

SATURDAY

SUNDAY

SHOPPING LIST

NOTES:

WEEKLY MEAL PLANNER

WEEK _______________   MONTH _______________

MONDAY

SATURDAY

TUESDAY

SUNDAY

WEDNESDAY

SHOPPING LIST

THURSDAY

FRIDAY

NOTES:

WEEKLY MEAL PLANNER

WEEK _______________   MONTH _______________

MONDAY

SATURDAY

TUESDAY

SUNDAY

WEDNESDAY

SHOPPING LIST

THURSDAY

FRIDAY

NOTES:

WEEKLY MEAL PLANNER

WEEK _______________   MONTH _______________

MONDAY

SATURDAY

TUESDAY

SUNDAY

WEDNESDAY

SHOPPING LIST

THURSDAY

FRIDAY

NOTES:

WEEKLY MEAL PLANNER

WEEK ________________   MONTH ________________

MONDAY

SATURDAY

TUESDAY

SUNDAY

WEDNESDAY

SHOPPING LIST

THURSDAY

FRIDAY

NOTES:

WEEKLY MEAL PLANNER

WEEK _______________   MONTH _______________

MONDAY

SATURDAY

TUESDAY

SUNDAY

WEDNESDAY

SHOPPING LIST

THURSDAY

FRIDAY

NOTES:

WEEKLY MEAL PLANNER

WEEK _______________________   MONTH _______________________

MONDAY

SATURDAY

TUESDAY

SUNDAY

WEDNESDAY

SHOPPING LIST

THURSDAY

FRIDAY

NOTES:

WEEKLY MEAL PLANNER

WEEK ___________________   MONTH ___________________

MONDAY

SATURDAY

TUESDAY

SUNDAY

WEDNESDAY

SHOPPING LIST

THURSDAY

FRIDAY

NOTES:

WEEKLY MEAL PLANNER

WEEK _______________ MONTH _______________

MONDAY

SATURDAY

TUESDAY

SUNDAY

WEDNESDAY

SHOPPING LIST

THURSDAY

FRIDAY

NOTES:

WEEK ——————— MONTH ———————

WEEKLY MEAL PLANNER

WEEK ______________________   MONTH ______________________

MONDAY

SATURDAY

TUESDAY

SUNDAY

WEDNESDAY

SHOPPING LIST

THURSDAY

FRIDAY

NOTES:

WEEKLY MEAL PLANNER

WEEK __________________   MONTH __________________

MONDAY

TUESDAY

WEDNESDAY

THURSDAY

FRIDAY

SATURDAY

SUNDAY

SHOPPING LIST

-
-
-
-
-
-
-
-

NOTES:

-
-
-
-

WEEKLY MEAL PLANNER

WEEK ___________________   MONTH ___________________

MONDAY

SATURDAY

TUESDAY

SUNDAY

WEDNESDAY

SHOPPING LIST

- ___________________
- ___________________
- ___________________
- ___________________
- ___________________
- ___________________
- ___________________
- ___________________

THURSDAY

FRIDAY

NOTES:

- ___________________
- ___________________
- ___________________
- ___________________